Today, eat smaller portions and exercise.

YOU ABSOLUTELY *CAN* DO THIS!

Today, eat less food and exercise.

YOU ABSOLUTELY *CAN* DO THIS!

INTRODUCTION

Think about it. How many scam weight loss diets, nutritional supplements and exercise contraptions have you heard advertised over the last, oh, *forever* number of years. They all represent to be "the one" that truly works because of the newfangled foo-foo dust du jour that they recently discovered (uh, yeah) enables one to lose weight, and keep it off, with little to no effort on your part. Seriously, if I had a nickle for every time I heard, read or was told about such a scam, I'd be richer than that Warren Buffet character. Speaking of which, this guy really cracks me up. He owns a UUUUUUGE, as the Donald would say, stake in Coca-Cola which he's owned forever. This company's business model is to get you to drink, and get hooked on, fizzy sugar water that costs pennies to make, and millions if not billions to recover from.

Everyone knows, which speaks volumes of the intelligence level of people around the globe, that not only does fizzy sugar water, also known as soda, have absolutely positively no redeeming nutritional level whatsoever, but it is down right, unequivocally and scientifically proven to be extremely BAD for you. No one, with even an eighth of a brain in their head, will argue this point. Yet people around the world continue to consume YUUUUUUUGE quantities of this potentially deadly substance, on a daily basis. This moronic act makes Mr. Buffet and his company A LOT of money.

Yet this YUUUUUUUGE (I just love saying and spelling this Donald Trumpism) amount of money made off of the stupidity of people is not enough for Mr. Buffet. On the contrary, he also is making money off of these people AFTER they get sick from drinking this crap (pardon my French). You see, science and the medical community have also shown, indisputably, that obesity is one of the primary causes of kidney failure. This is because obesity typically leads to diabetes and high blood pressure, which in turn cause one's kidneys to fail. By drinking fizzy sugar water, the sugar consumed is converted into fat and stored in your body, causing you to become obese. This in turn is likely to make you diabetic and cause you to develop high blood pressure which may lead to your kidneys failing. And this is where the vaunted Mr. Buffet will make more money off of your slowly dying, soon to be corpse. How, can this be so you may ask yourself. Well, Mr. Buffet, being the astute investor that he is, has also invested YUUUUUUUGE in a company that owns kidney dialysis clinics all across the country. Hence, the more fizzy sugar water poison you drink, the more money Mr. Buffet makes. Then, after you've drank enough of the poison to make you obese, diabetic and prone to high blood pressure, Mr. Buffet will then make another fortune once your kidneys fail. This guy truly is good at making money!

Now, enough about Mr. Buffet and back to the matter at hand, namely, healthy weight loss. Before we get into the nuts and bolts of healthy weight loss, I first want to talk about habit formation. In 1960, a plastic surgeon by the name Maxwell Maltz published a book called *Psycho-Cymbernetics* that dealt with behavior change. In that book, Dr. Maltz talked about his observations of how long it typically took his patients to become comfortable with a procedure they had done, whether that procedure was a nose, for example, or an amputated limb. He concluded that it took at least 21 days before a patient adjusted to their situation. He also observed that it took himself at least 21 days to form a new habit.

Over the years, many self-help gurus took this reference from Dr. Maltz's book and began to preach that it takes 21 days to form a new habit, conveniently leaving out the phrase "a minimum of about..." before "21 days." Thus, the myth of it taking 21 days to form a new habit was born. Years later, a health psychology researcher at University College London, Phillippa Lally, and her team performed a study to determine how long it actually takes to form a habit. They studied 96 people over a 12 week period and concluded that, **on average**, it takes more than two months before a new behavior becomes automatic, or to be more precise, 66 days. Though the study found the time period for forming a new habit to be between 18 and 254 days, the **average** was 66 days.

This now brings us to the nuts and bolts of this book which, as the title proclaims, "healthy weight loss guaranteed, or your money back". By reading the following pages every day (its OK to skip a day here or there without sabotaging yourself), one page per day, and truly taking the words to heart, your reward will be healthy weight loss that should last you a lifetime. Good luck and know that I'm rooting for you!

Today, eat less food and workout.

YOU ABSOLUTELY *CAN* DO THIS!

Today, watch your food intake and exercise.

YOU ABSOLUTELY *CAN* DO THIS!

Today, watch your food intake and do something aerobic.

YOU ABSOLUTELY *CAN* DO THIS!

Today, watch how much you eat and do something aerobic.

YOU ABSOLUTELY *CAN* DO THIS!

Today, watch how much you eat and do something anaerobic.

YOU ABSOLUTELY *CAN* DO THIS!

Today, eat less than normal and exercise.

YOU ABSOLUTELY *CAN* DO THIS!

Today, eat less than normal and get your heart rate up by moving around.

YOU ABSOLUTELY *CAN* DO THIS!

Today, be mindful of how much you eat and get your heart rate up by moving around.

YOU ABSOLUTELY *CAN* DO THIS!

Today, be the master of your appetite and lift some weights.

YOU ABSOLUTELY *CAN* DO THIS!

Today, do not overeat and do something physical.

YOU ABSOLUTELY *CAN* DO THIS!

Today, watch what, and how much you eat and do something physical.

YOU ABSOLUTELY *CAN* DO THIS!

Today, eat less and do not forget to exercise.

YOU ABSOLUTELY *CAN* DO THIS!

Today, eat only until you feel full and do something physical.

YOU ABSOLUTELY *CAN* DO THIS!

Today, eat only until you feel full and get in some exercise.

YOU ABSOLUTELY *CAN* DO THIS!

Today, eat smaller portions and exercise.

DO THIS FOR **YOU**!

Today, eat less food and exercise.

DO THIS FOR **YOU**!

Today, eat less food and workout.

DO THIS FOR **YOU**!

Today, watch your food intake and exercise.

DO THIS FOR **YOU**!

Today, watch your food intake and do something aerobic.

DO THIS FOR **YOU**!

Today, watch how much you eat and do something aerobic.

DO THIS FOR **YOU**!

Today, watch how much you eat and do something anaerobic.

DO THIS FOR **YOU**!

Today, eat less than normal and exercise.

DO THIS FOR **YOU**!

Today, eat less than normal and get your heart rate up by moving around.

DO THIS FOR **YOU**!

Today, be mindful of how much you eat and get your heart rate up by moving around.

DO THIS FOR **YOU**!

Today, be the master of your appetite and lift some weights.

DO THIS FOR **YOU**!

Today, do not overeat and do something physical.

DO THIS FOR **YOU**!

Today, eat less and do not forget to exercise.

DO THIS FOR **YOU**!

Today, eat only until you feel full and do something physical.

DO THIS FOR **YOU**!

Today, eat only until you feel full and do something to get your heart rate up.

DO THIS FOR **YOU**!

Today, eat smaller portions and exercise.

YOU ARE WORTH IT!

Today, eat less food and exercise.

YOU ARE WORTH IT!

Today, eat less food and workout.

YOU ARE WORTH IT!

Today, watch your food intake and exercise.

YOU ARE WORTH IT!

Today, watch your food intake and do something aerobic.

YOU ARE WORTH IT!

Today, watch how much you eat and do something aerobic.

YOU ARE WORTH IT!

Today, watch how much you eat and do something anaerobic.

YOU ARE WORTH IT!

Today, eat less than normal and exercise.

YOU ARE WORTH IT!

Today, eat less than normal and get your heart rate up by moving around.

YOU ARE WORTH IT!

Today, be mindful of how much you eat and get your heart rate up by moving around.

YOU ARE WORTH IT!

Today, be the master of your appetite and lift some weights.

YOU ARE WORTH IT!

Today, do not overeat and do something physical.

YOU ARE WORTH IT!

Today, eat less and do not forget to exercise.

YOU ARE WORTH IT!

Today, eat only until you feel full and do something physical.

YOU ARE WORTH IT!

Today, eat only until you feel full and do something to get your heart rate up.

YOU ARE WORTH IT!

Today, eat smaller portions and exercise.

LOVE **YOURSELF**!

Today, eat less food and exercise.

LOVE **YOURSELF**!

Today, eat less food and workout.

LOVE **YOURSELF**!

Today, watch your food intake and exercise.

LOVE **YOURSELF**!

Today, watch your food intake and do something aerobic.

LOVE **YOURSELF**!

Today, watch how much you eat and do something aerobic.

LOVE **YOURSELF**!

Today, watch how much you eat and do something anaerobic.

LOVE **YOURSELF**!

Today, eat less than normal and exercise.

LOVE **YOURSELF**!

Today, eat less than normal and get your heart rate up by moving around.

LOVE **YOURSELF**!

Today, be mindful of how much you eat and get your heart rate up by moving around.

LOVE **YOURSELF**!

Today, be the master of your appetite and lift some weights.

LOVE **YOURSELF**!

Today, do not overeat and do something physical.

LOVE **YOURSELF**!

Today, eat less and do not forget to exercise.

LOVE **YOURSELF**!

Today, eat only until you feel full and do something physical.

LOVE **YOURSELF**!

Today, eat only until you feel full and do something to get your heart rate up.

LOVE **YOURSELF**!

Today, eat less food and exercise.

CONGRATULATIONS!

Today, eat less food and workout.

YOU DID IT!

Today, watch your food intake and exercise.

SUCCESS!

Today, watch your food intake and do something aerobic.

YES!

Today, watch how much you eat and do something aerobic.

YOU ARE *THE BEST*!

By now, eating less and exercising should be a newly formed habit. If not, go back to day 1 and re-read the pages. You may need some added repetition for the new habit to fully set in.

As I stated in the introduction to the book, there are no magic potions, pills, elixirs, supplements or devices for achieving healthy and sustainable weight loss. Only eating less and exercise can yield this result. These are lifestyle changes, not quick-fix, one-off gimmicks.

Now, if you can look yourself in the mirror and say that you honestly adhered to the mantras in this book but somehow still failed to lose weight, I will refund you the cost of the book and strongly recommend that you see a medical professional for you may have a serious health problem, all kidding aside.

www.ingramcontent.com/pod-product-compliance
Lightning Source LLC
Chambersburg PA
CBHW062019280526
45787CB00005B/2159